This Book Belongs To:

____

My Table Of Contents:

Page	Product Name	Rating /5	Favorites
1			
2			
3			
4			
5			
6			
7			
8			
9			
10			
11			
12			
13			
14			
15			
16			
17			
18			
19			
20			
21			
22			
23			
24			
25			
26			
27			
28			

Add the products you love to the "favorites" column

My Table Of Contents:

Page	Product Name	Rating /5	Favorites
29			
30			
31			
32			
33			
34			
35			
36			
37			
38			
39			
40			
41			
42			
43			
44			
45			
46			
47			
48			
49			
50			
51			
52			
53			
54	Product Name	Rating /5	Favorites
55			
56			

My Table Of Contents:

Page	Product Name	Rating /5	Favorites
57			
58			
59			
60			
61			
62			
63			
64			
65			
66			
67			
68			
69			
70			
71			
72			
73			
74			
75			
76			
77			
78			
79			
80			
81			
82			
83			
84			

My Table Of Contents:

Page	Product Name	Rating /5	Favorites
85			
86			
87			
88			
89			
90			
91			
92			
93			
94			
95			
96			
97			
98			
99			
100			
101			
102			
103			
104			
105			
106			
107			
108			
109			
110			

Product Name:	Price:

Descript on:

"Good" Ingredients:

"Bad" Ingredients:

Pros:

Cons:

Would I repurchase?

Would I recommend it?

RATING: ☆ ☆ ☆ ☆ ☆

Detailed review and additional notes:

Date:

Product Name:	Price:

Description:

"Good" Ingredients:

"Bad" Ingredients:

Pros:

Cons:

Would I repurchase?

Would I recommend it?

RATING: ☆ ☆ ☆ ☆ ☆

Detailed review and additional notes:

Date:

Product Name:	Price:

Description:

"Good" Ingredients:

"Bad" Ingredients:

Pros:

Cons:

Would I repurchase?

Would I recommend it?

RATING: ☆ ☆ ☆ ☆ ☆

Detailed review and additional notes:

Date:

Product Name:	Price:

Description:

"Good" Ingredients:

"Bad" Ingredients:

Pros:

Cons:

Would I repurchase?
Would I recommend it?

RATING: ☆ ☆ ☆ ☆ ☆

Detailed review and additional notes:

Date:

Product Name:	Price:
Description:	
"Good" Ingredients:	
"Bad" Ingredients:	
Pros:	
Cons:	
Would I repurchase?	
Would I recommend it?	

RATING: ☆ ☆ ☆ ☆ ☆

Detailed review and additional notes:

Date:

Product Name:	Price:

Description:

"Good" Ingredients:

"Bad" Ingredients:

Pros:

Cons:

Would I repurchase?

Would I recommend it?

RATING: ☆ ☆ ☆ ☆ ☆

Detailed review and additional notes:

Date:

Product Name:	Price:

Descript on:

"Good" Ingredients:

"Bad" Ingredients:

Pros:

Cons:

Would I repurchase?

Would I recommend it?

RATING: ☆ ☆ ☆ ☆ ☆

Detailed review and additional notes:

Date:

Product Name:	Price:

Description:

"Good" Ingredients:

"Bad" Ingredients:

Pros:

Cons:

Would I repurchase?

Would I recommend it?

RATING: ☆ ☆ ☆ ☆ ☆

Detailed review and additional notes:

Date:

Product Name:	Price:

Description:

"Good" ngredients:

"Bad" Ingredients:

Pros:

Cons:

Would I repurchase?

Would I recommend it?

RATING: ☆ ☆ ☆ ☆ ☆

Detailec review and additional notes:

Date:

Product Name:	Price:

Description:

"Good" Ingredients:

"Bad" Ingredients:

Pros:

Cons:

Would I repurchase?

Would I recommend it?

RATING: ☆ ☆ ☆ ☆ ☆

Detailed review and additional notes:

Date:

Product Name:	Price:

Description:

"Good" Ingredients:

"Bad" Ingredients:

Pros:

Cons:

Would I repurchase?

Would I recommend it?

RATING: ☆ ☆ ☆ ☆ ☆

Detailed review and additional notes:

Date:

Product Name:	Price:
Description:	
"Good" Ingredients:	
"Bad" Ingredients:	
Pros:	
Cons:	

Would I repurchase?

Would I recommend it?

RATING: ☆ ☆ ☆ ☆ ☆

Detailed review and additional notes:

Date:

Product Name:	Price:

Descript on:

"Good" Ingredients:

"Bad" Ingredients:

Pros:

Cons:

Would I repurchase?

Would I recommend it?

RATING: ☆ ☆ ☆ ☆ ☆

Detailed review and additional notes:

Date:

Product Name:	Price:

Description:

"Good" Ingredients:

"Bad" Ingredients:

Pros:

Cons:

Would I repurchase?

Would I recommend it?

RATING: ☆ ☆ ☆ ☆ ☆

Detailed review and additional notes:

Date:

Product Name:	Price:

Description:

"Good" Ingredients:

"Bad" Ingredients:

Pros:

Cons:

Would I repurchase?

Would I recommend it?

RATING: ☆ ☆ ☆ ☆ ☆

Detailed review and additional notes:

Product Name:	Price:

Description:

"Good" Ingredients:

"Bad" Ingredients:

Pros:

Cons:

Would I repurchase?
Would I recommend it?

RATING: ☆ ☆ ☆ ☆ ☆

Detailed review and additional notes:

Date:

Product Name:	Price:

Description:

"Good" Ingredients:

"Bad" Ingredients:

Pros:

Cons:

Would I repurchase?

Would I recommend it?

RATING: ☆ ☆ ☆ ☆ ☆

Detailed review and additional notes:

Date:

Product Name:	Price:

Description:

"Good" Ingredients:

"Bad" Ingredients:

Pros:

Cons:

Would I repurchase?

Would I recommend it?

RATING: ☆ ☆ ☆ ☆ ☆

Detailed review and additional notes:

Date:

Product Name:	Price:

Description:

"Good" Ingredients:

"Bad" Ingredients:

Pros:

Cons:

Would I repurchase?

Would I recommend it?

RATING: ☆ ☆ ☆ ☆ ☆

Detailed review and additional notes:

Date:

Product Name:	Price:

Description:

"Good" Ingredients:

"Bad" Ingredients:

Pros:

Cons:

Would I repurchase?

Would I recommend it?

RATING: ☆ ☆ ☆ ☆ ☆

Detailed review and additional notes:

Date:

Product Name:	Price:

Description:

"Good" ngredients:

"Bad" Ingredients:

Pros:

Cons:

Would I repurchase?

Would I recommend it?

RATING: ☆ ☆ ☆ ☆ ☆

Detailec review and additional notes:

Date:

Product Name:	Price:

Description:

"Good" Ingredients:

"Bad" Ingredients:

Pros:

Cons:

Would I repurchase?

Would I recommend it?

RATING: ☆ ☆ ☆ ☆ ☆

Detailed review and additional notes:

Product Name:	Price:

Description:

"Good" Ingredients:

"Bad" Ingredients:

Pros:

Cons:

Would I repurchase?

Would I recommend it?

RATING: ☆ ☆ ☆ ☆ ☆

Detailed review and additional notes:

Date:

Product Name:	Price:

Description:

"Good" Ingredients:

"Bad" Ingredients:

Pros:

Cons:

Would I repurchase?

Would I recommend it?

RATING: ☆ ☆ ☆ ☆ ☆

Detailed review and additional notes:

Date:

Product Name:	Price:

Description:

"Good" Ingredients:

"Bad" Ingredients:

Pros:

Cons:

Would I repurchase?

Would I recommend it?

RATING: ☆ ☆ ☆ ☆ ☆

Detailed review and additional notes:

Date:

Product Name:	Price:

Description:

"Good" Ingredients:

"Bad" Ingredients:

Pros:

Cons:

Would I repurchase?

Would I recommend it?

RATING: ☆ ☆ ☆ ☆ ☆

Detailed review and additional notes:

Date:

Product Name:	Price:

Description:

"Good" Ingredients:

"Bad" Ingredients:

Pros:

Cons:

Would I repurchase?

Would I recommend it?

RATING: ☆ ☆ ☆ ☆ ☆

Detailed review and additional notes:

Date:

Product Name:	Price:

Description:

"Good" Ingredients:

"Bad" Ingredients:

Pros:

Cons:

Would I repurchase?
Would I recommend it?

RATING: ☆ ☆ ☆ ☆ ☆

Detailed review and additional notes:

Date:

Product Name:	Price:

Description:

"Good" Ingredients:

"Bad" Ingredients:

Pros:

Cons:

Would I repurchase?

Would I recommend it?

RATING: ☆ ☆ ☆ ☆ ☆

Detailed review and additional notes:

Date:

Product Name:	Price:

Description:

"Good" Ingredients:

"Bad" Ingredients:

Pros:

Cons:

Would I repurchase?

Would I recommend it?

RATING: ☆ ☆ ☆ ☆ ☆

Detailed review and additional notes:

Date:

Product Name:	Price:

Descript on:

"Good" Ingredients:

"Bad" Ingredients:

Pros:

Cons:

Would I repurchase?

Would I recommend it?

RATING: ☆ ☆ ☆ ☆ ☆

Detailed review and additional notes:

Date:

Product Name:	Price:

Description:

"Good" Ingredients:

"Bad" Ingredients:

Pros:

Cons:

Would I repurchase?

Would I recommend it?

RATING: ☆ ☆ ☆ ☆ ☆

Detailed review and additional notes:

Date:

Product Name:	Price:

Description:

"Good" Ingredients:

"Bad" Ingredients:

Pros:

Cons:

Would I repurchase?

Would I recommend it?

RATING: ☆ ☆ ☆ ☆ ☆

Detailed review and additional notes:

Date:

Product Name:	Price:

Description:

"Good" Ingredients:

"Bad" Ingredients:

Pros:

Cons:

Would I repurchase?

Would I recommend it?

RATING: ☆ ☆ ☆ ☆ ☆

Detailed review and additional notes:

Date:

| Product Name: | Price: |

Description:

"Good" Ingredients:

"Bad" Ingredients:

Pros:

Cons:

Would I repurchase?

Would I recommend it?

RATING: ☆ ☆ ☆ ☆ ☆

Detailed review and additional notes:

Date:

Product Name:	Price:

Description:

"Good" Ingredients:

"Bad" Ingredients:

Pros:

Cons:

Would I repurchase?

Would I recommend it?

RATING: ☆ ☆ ☆ ☆ ☆

Detailed review and additional notes:

Date:

Product Name:	Price:

Descript on:

"Good" Ingredients:

"Bad" Ingredients:

Pros:

Cons:

Would I repurchase?

Would I recommend it?

RATING: ☆ ☆ ☆ ☆ ☆

Detailed review and additional notes:

Date:

Product Name:	Price:

Description:

"Good" Ingredients:

"Bad" Ingredients:

Pros:

Cons:

Would I repurchase?

Would I recommend it?

RATING: ☆ ☆ ☆ ☆ ☆

Detailed review and additional notes:

Date:

Product Name:	Price:

Description:

"Good" Ingredients:

"Bad" Ingredients:

Pros:

Cons:

Would I repurchase?

Would I recommend it?

RATING: ☆ ☆ ☆ ☆ ☆

Detailed review and additional notes:

Date:

Product Name:	Price:

Description:

"Good" Ingredients:

"Bad" Ingredients:

Pros:

Cons:

Would I repurchase?

Would I recommend it?

RATING: ☆ ☆ ☆ ☆ ☆

Detailed review and additional notes:

Date:

Product Name:	Price:

Description:

"Good" Ingredients:

"Bad" Ingredients:

Pros:

Cons:

Would I repurchase?

Would I recommend it?

RATING: ☆ ☆ ☆ ☆ ☆

Detailed review and additional notes:

Date:

Product Name:	Price:

Description:

"Good" Ingredients:

"Bad" Ingredients:

Pros:

Cons:

Would I repurchase?

Would I recommend it?

RATING: ☆ ☆ ☆ ☆ ☆

Detailed review and additional notes:

Date:

Product Name:	Price:

Description:

"Good" Ingredients:

"Bad" Ingredients:

Pros:

Cons:

Would I repurchase?

Would I recommend it?

RATING: ☆ ☆ ☆ ☆ ☆

Detailed review and additional notes:

Date:

Product Name:	Price:

Description:

"Good" Ingredients:

"Bad" Ingredients:

Pros:

Cons:

Would I repurchase?

Would I recommend it?

RATING: ☆ ☆ ☆ ☆ ☆

Detailed review and additional notes:

Date:

Product Name:	Price:

Description:

"Good" Ingredients:

"Bad" Ingredients:

Pros:

Cons:

Would I repurchase?

Would I recommend it?

RATING: ☆ ☆ ☆ ☆ ☆

Detailed review and additional notes:

Product Name:	Price:

Description:

"Good" Ingredients:

"Bad" Ingredients:

Pros:

Cons:

Would I repurchase?

Would I recommend it?

RATING: ☆ ☆ ☆ ☆ ☆

Detailed review and additional notes:

Date:

Product Name:	Price:

Description:

"Good" Ingredients:

"Bad" Ingredients:

Pros:

Cons:

Would I repurchase?

Would I recommend it?

RATING: ☆ ☆ ☆ ☆ ☆

Detailed review and additional notes:

Date:

Product Name:	Price:

Description:

"Good" Ingredients:

"Bad" Ingredients:

Pros:

Cons:

Would I repurchase?

Would I recommend it?

RATING: ☆ ☆ ☆ ☆ ☆

Detailed review and additional notes:

Date:

Product Name:	Price:

Description:

"Good" Ingredients:

"Bad" Ingredients:

Pros:

Cons:

Would I repurchase?

Would I recommend it?

RATING: ☆ ☆ ☆ ☆ ☆

Detailed review and additional notes:

Date:

Product Name:	Price:

Description:

"Good" Ingredients:

"Bad" Ingredients:

Pros:

Cons:

Would I repurchase?

Would I recommend it?

RATING: ☆ ☆ ☆ ☆ ☆

Detailed review and additional notes:

Date:

Product Name:	Price:

Description:

"Good" Ingredients:

"Bad" Ingredients:

Pros:

Cons:

Would I repurchase?

Would I recommend it?

RATING: ☆ ☆ ☆ ☆ ☆

Detailed review and additional notes:

Date:

Product Name:	Price:

Description:

"Good" Ingredients:

"Bad" Ingredients:

Pros:

Cons:

Would I repurchase?

Would I recommend it?

RATING: ☆ ☆ ☆ ☆ ☆

Detailed review and additional notes:

Date:

Product Name:	Price:

Description:

"Good" Ingredients:

"Bad" Ingredients:

Pros:

Cons:

Would I repurchase?

Would I recommend it?

RATING: ☆ ☆ ☆ ☆ ☆

Detailed review and additional notes:

Date:

Product Name:	Price:

Description:

"Good" Ingredients:

"Bad" Ingredients:

Pros:

Cons:

Would I repurchase?

Would I recommend it?

RATING: ☆ ☆ ☆ ☆ ☆

Detailed review and additional notes:

Date:

Product Name:	Price:

Description:

"Good" Ingredients:

"Bad" Ingredients:

Pros:

Cons:

Would I repurchase?

Would I recommend it?

RATING: ☆ ☆ ☆ ☆ ☆

Detailed review and additional notes:

Date:

Product Name:	Price:

Description:

"Good" Ingredients:

"Bad" Ingredients:

Pros:

Cons:

Would I repurchase?

Would I recommend it?

RATING: ☆ ☆ ☆ ☆ ☆

Detailed review and additional notes:

Product Name:	Price:

Description:

"Good" Ingredients:

"Bad" Ingredients:

Pros:

Cons:

Would I repurchase?

Would I recommend it?

RATING: ☆ ☆ ☆ ☆ ☆

Detailed review and additional notes:

Date:

Product Name:	Price:

Description:

"Good" Ingredients:

"Bad" Ingredients:

Pros:

Cons:

Would I repurchase?

Would I recommend it?

RATING: ☆ ☆ ☆ ☆ ☆

Detailed review and additional notes:

Date:

Product Name:	Price:

Description:

"Good" Ingredients:

"Bad" Ingredients:

Pros:

Cons:

Would I repurchase?

Would I recommend it?

RATING: ☆ ☆ ☆ ☆ ☆

Detailed review and additional notes:

Date:

Product Name:	Price:

Description:

"Good" Ingredients:

"Bad" Ingredients:

Pros:

Cons:

Would I repurchase?

Would I recommend it?

RATING: ☆ ☆ ☆ ☆ ☆

Detailed review and additional notes:

Date:

Product Name:	Price:

Description:

"Good" Ingredients:

"Bad" Ingredients:

Pros:

Cons:

Would I repurchase?

Would I recommend it?

RATING: ☆ ☆ ☆ ☆ ☆

Detailed review and additional notes:

Date:

Product Name:	Price:

Description:

"Good" Ingredients:

"Bad" Ingredients:

Pros:

Cons:

Would I repurchase?

Would I recommend it?

RATING: ☆ ☆ ☆ ☆ ☆

Detailed review and additional notes:

Date:

Product Name:	Price:

Description:

"Good" Ingredients:

"Bad" Ingredients:

Pros:

Cons:

Would I repurchase?

Would I recommend it?

RATING: ☆ ☆ ☆ ☆ ☆

Detailed review and additional notes:

Date:

Product Name:	Price:

Description:

"Good" Ingredients:

"Bad" Ingredients:

Pros:

Cons:

Would I repurchase?

Would I recommend it?

RATING: ☆ ☆ ☆ ☆ ☆

Detailed review and additional notes:

Date:

Product Name:	Price:

Description:

"Good" Ingredients:

"Bad" Ingredients:

Pros:

Cons:

Would I repurchase?

Would I recommend it?

RATING: ☆ ☆ ☆ ☆ ☆

Detailed review and additional notes:

Date:

| Product Name: | Price: |

Description:

"Good" Ingredients:

"Bad" Ingredients:

Pros:

Cons:

Would I repurchase?

Would I recommend it?

RATING: ☆ ☆ ☆ ☆ ☆

Detailed review and additional notes:

Date:

Product Name:	Price:

Description:

"Good" Ingredients:

"Bad" Ingredients:

Pros:

Cons:

Would I repurchase?

Would I recommend it?

RATING: ☆ ☆ ☆ ☆ ☆

Detailed review and additional notes:

Date:

Product Name:	Price:

Description:

"Good" Ingredients:

"Bad" Ingredients:

Pros:

Cons:

Would I repurchase?

Would I recommend it?

RATING: ☆ ☆ ☆ ☆ ☆

Detailed review and additional notes:

Date:

Product Name:	Price:

Description:

"Good" Ingredients:

"Bad" Ingredients:

Pros:

Cons:

Would I repurchase?

Would I recommend it?

RATING: ☆ ☆ ☆ ☆ ☆

Detailed review and additional notes:

Date:

Product Name:	Price:

Description:

"Good" Ingredients:

"Bad" Ingredients:

Pros:

Cons:

Would I repurchase?

Would I recommend it?

RATING: ☆ ☆ ☆ ☆ ☆

Detailed review and additional notes:

Date:

Product Name:	Price:

Description:

"Good" Ingredients:

"Bad" Ingredients:

Pros:

Cons:

Would I repurchase?

Would I recommend it?

RATING: ☆ ☆ ☆ ☆ ☆

Detailed review and additional notes:

Date:

Product Name:	Price:

Description:

"Good" Ingredients:

"Bad" Ingredients:

Pros:

Cons:

Would I repurchase?

Would I recommend it?

RATING: ☆ ☆ ☆ ☆ ☆

Detailed review and additional notes:

Date:

Product Name:	Price:

Description:

"Good" Ingredients:

"Bad" Ingredients:

Pros:

Cons:

Would I repurchase?

Would I recommend it?

RATING: ☆ ☆ ☆ ☆ ☆

Detailed review and additional notes:

Date:

Product Name:	Price:

Description:

"Good" Ingredients:

"Bad" Ingredients:

Pros:

Cons:

Would I repurchase?

Would I recommend it?

RATING: ☆ ☆ ☆ ☆ ☆

Detailed review and additional notes:

Date:

Product Name:	Price:

Description:

"Good" Ingredients:

"Bad" Ingredients:

Pros:

Cons:

Would I repurchase?

Would I recommend it?

RATING: ☆ ☆ ☆ ☆ ☆

Detailed review and additional notes:

Date:

Product Name:	Price:

Description:

"Good" Ingredients:

"Bad" Ingredients:

Pros:

Cons:

Would I repurchase?

Would I recommend it?

RATING: ☆ ☆ ☆ ☆ ☆

Detailed review and additional notes:

Date:

Product Name:	Price:

Description:

"Good" Ingredients:

"Bad" Ingredients:

Pros:

Cons:

Would I repurchase?

Would I recommend it?

RATING: ☆ ☆ ☆ ☆ ☆

Detailed review and additional notes:

Date:

Product Name:	Price:

Description:

"Good" Ingredients:

"Bad" Ingredients:

Pros:

Cons:

Would I repurchase?

Would I recommend it?

RATING: ☆ ☆ ☆ ☆ ☆

Detailed review and additional notes:

Date:

Product Name:	Price:

Description:

"Good" Ingredients:

"Bad" Ingredients:

Pros:

Cons:

Would I repurchase?

Would I recommend it?

RATING: ☆ ☆ ☆ ☆ ☆

Detailed review and additional notes:

Date:

Product Name:	Price:

Description:

"Good" Ingredients:

"Bad" Ingredients:

Pros:

Cons:

Would I repurchase?

Would I recommend it?

RATING: ☆ ☆ ☆ ☆ ☆

Detailed review and additional notes:

Date:

Product Name:	Price:

Description:

"Good" Ingredients:

"Bad" Ingredients:

Pros:

Cons:

Would I repurchase?

Would I recommend it?

RATING: ☆ ☆ ☆ ☆ ☆

Detailed review and additional notes:

Date:

Product Name:	Price:

Description:

"Good" Ingredients:

"Bad" Ingredients:

Pros:

Cons:

Would I repurchase?

Would I recommend it?

RATING: ☆ ☆ ☆ ☆ ☆

Detailed review and additional notes:

Date:

Product Name:	Price:

Description:

"Good" Ingredients:

"Bad" Ingredients:

Pros:

Cons:

Would I repurchase?

Would I recommend it?

RATING: ☆ ☆ ☆ ☆ ☆

Detailed review and additional notes:

Date:

Product Name:	Price:

Description:

"Good" Ingredients:

"Bad" Ingredients:

Pros:

Cons:

Would I repurchase?

Would I recommend it?

RATING: ☆ ☆ ☆ ☆ ☆

Detailed review and additional notes:

Date:

Product Name:	Price:

Description:

"Good" Ingredients:

"Bad" Ingredients:

Pros:

Cons:

Would I repurchase?

Would I recommend it?

RATING: ☆ ☆ ☆ ☆ ☆

Detailed review and additional notes:

Product Name:	Price:

Description:

"Good" Ingredients:

"Bad" Ingredients:

Pros:

Cons:

Would I repurchase?

Would I recommend it?

RATING: ☆ ☆ ☆ ☆ ☆

Detailed review and additional notes:

Date:

Product Name:	Price:

Description:

"Good" Ingredients:

"Bad" Ingredients:

Pros:

Cons:

Would I repurchase?

Would I recommend it?

RATING: ☆ ☆ ☆ ☆ ☆

Detailed review and additional notes:

Date:

Product Name:	Price:

Description:

"Good" Ingredients:

"Bad" Ingredients:

Pros:

Cons:

Would I repurchase?

Would I recommend it?

RATING: ☆ ☆ ☆ ☆ ☆

Detailed review and additional notes:

Date:

Product Name:	Price:

Description:

"Good" Ingredients:

"Bad" Ingredients:

Pros:

Cons:

Would I repurchase?

Would I recommend it?

RATING: ☆ ☆ ☆ ☆ ☆

Detailed review and additional notes:

Date:

Product Name:	Price:

Description:

"Good" Ingredients:

"Bad" Ingredients:

Pros:

Cons:

Would I repurchase?

Would I recommend it?

RATING: ☆ ☆ ☆ ☆ ☆

Detailed review and additional notes:

Date:

| Product Name: | Price: |

Description:

"Good" Ingredients:

"Bad" Ingredients:

Pros:

Cons:

Would I repurchase?

Would I recommend it?

RATING: ☆ ☆ ☆ ☆ ☆

Detailed review and additional notes:

Date:

Product Name:	Price:

Description:

"Good" Ingredients:

"Bad" Ingredients:

Pros:

Cons:

Would I repurchase?

Would I recommend it?

RATING: ☆ ☆ ☆ ☆ ☆

Detailed review and additional notes:

Date:

Product Name:	Price:

Descript on:

"Good" Ingredients:

"Bad" Ingredients:

Pros:

Cons:

Would I repurchase?

Would I recommend it?

RATING: ☆ ☆ ☆ ☆ ☆

Detailed review and additional notes:

Date:

Product Name:	Price:

Description:

"Good" Ingredients:

"Bad" Ingredients:

Pros:

Cons:

Would I repurchase?

Would I recommend it?

RATING: ☆ ☆ ☆ ☆ ☆

Detailed review and additional notes:

Date:

Product Name:	Price:

Description:

"Good" Ingredients:

"Bad" Ingredients:

Pros:

Cons:

Would I repurchase?

Would I recommend it?

RATING: ☆ ☆ ☆ ☆ ☆

Detailed review and additional notes:

Date:

Product Name:	Price:

Description:

"Good" Ingredients:

"Bad" Ingredients:

Pros:

Cons:

Would I repurchase?

Would I recommend it?

RATING: ☆ ☆ ☆ ☆ ☆

Detailed review and additional notes:

Date:

Product Name:	Price:

Description:

"Good" Ingredients:

"Bad" Ingredients:

Pros:

Cons:

Would I repurchase?

Would I recommend it?

RATING: ☆ ☆ ☆ ☆ ☆

Detailed review and additional notes:

Date:

Product Name:	Price:

Description:

"Good" Ingredients:

"Bad" Ingredients:

Pros:

Cons:

Would I repurchase?

Would I recommend it?

RATING: ☆ ☆ ☆ ☆ ☆

Detailed review and additional notes:

Date:

Product Name:	Price:

Description:

"Good" Ingredients:

"Bad" Ingredients:

Pros:

Cons:

Would I repurchase?

Would I recommend it?

RATING: ☆ ☆ ☆ ☆ ☆

Detailed review and additional notes:

Date:

Product Name:	Price:

Description:

"Good" Ingredients:

"Bad" Ingredients:

Pros:

Cons:

Would I repurchase?

Would I recommend it?

RATING: ☆ ☆ ☆ ☆ ☆

Detailed review and additional notes:

Date:

Product Name:	Price:

Description:

"Good" Ingredients:

"Bad" Ingredients:

Pros:

Cons:

Would I repurchase?

Would I recommend it?

RATING: ☆ ☆ ☆ ☆ ☆

Detailed review and additional notes:

Date:

Product Name:	Price:

Description:

"Good" Ingredients:

"Bad" Ingredients:

Pros:

Cons:

Would I repurchase?

Would I recommend it?

RATING: ☆ ☆ ☆ ☆ ☆

Detailed review and additional notes:

Date:

Product Name:	Price:

Description:

"Good" Ingredients:

"Bad" Ingredients:

Pros:

Cons:

Would I repurchase?

Would I recommend it?

RATING: ☆ ☆ ☆ ☆ ☆

Detailed review and additional notes:

Date:

Product Name:	Price:

Description:

"Good" Ingredients:

"Bad" Ingredients:

Pros:

Cons:

Would I repurchase?

Would I recommend it?

RATING: ☆ ☆ ☆ ☆ ☆

Detailed review and additional notes:

Date:

| Product Name: | Price: |

Description:

"Good" Ingredients:

"Bad" Ingredients:

Pros:

Cons:

Would I repurchase?

Would I recommend it?

RATING: ☆ ☆ ☆ ☆ ☆

Detailed review and additional notes:

Date:

Product Name:	Price:

Description:

"Good" Ingredients:

"Bad" Ingredients:

Pros:

Cons:

Would I repurchase?

Would I recommend it?

RATING: ☆ ☆ ☆ ☆ ☆

Detailed review and additional notes:

Date:

Product Name:	Price:

Description:

"Good" Ingredients:

"Bad" Ingredients:

Pros:

Cons:

Would I repurchase?

Would I recommend it?

RATING: ☆ ☆ ☆ ☆ ☆

Detailed review and additional notes:

Date:

Product Name:	Price:

Description:

"Good" Ingredients:

"Bad" Ingredients:

Pros:

Cons:

Would I repurchase?

Would I recommend it?

RATING: ☆ ☆ ☆ ☆ ☆

Detailed review and additional notes:

Date:

Product Name:	Price:

Description:

"Good" Ingredients:

"Bad" Ingredients:

Pros:

Cons:

Would I repurchase?

Would I recommend it?

RATING: ☆ ☆ ☆ ☆ ☆

Detailed review and additional notes:

Date:

Product Name:	Price:

Description:

"Good" Ingredients:

"Bad" Ingredients:

Pros:

Cons:

Would I repurchase?

Would I recommend it?

RATING: ☆ ☆ ☆ ☆ ☆

Detailed review and additional notes:

Notes

Notes

Notes

Notes

Notes